I0421527

Weight Loss

Coping with Obsessive Weight Watching

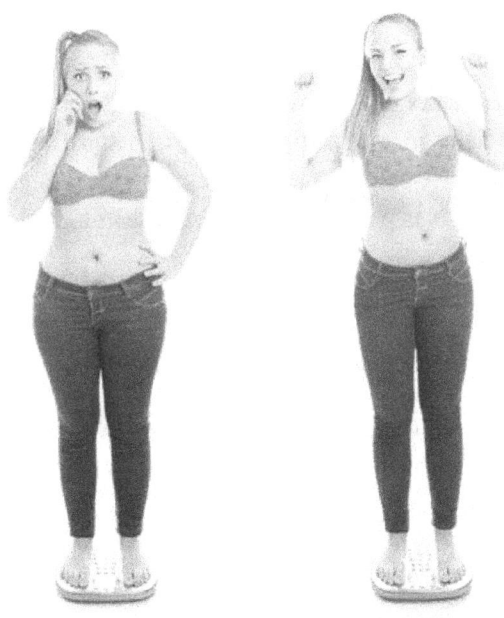

Dueep Jyot Singh

Mendon Cottage Books

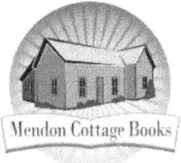

JD-Biz Publishing

Disclaimer

The information is this book is provided for informational purposes only. It is not intended to be used and medical advice or a substitute for proper medical treatment by a qualified health care provider. The information is believed to be accurate as presented based on research by the author.

The contents have not been evaluated by the U.S. Food and Drug Administration or any other Government or Health Organization and the contents in this book are not to be used to treat cure or prevent disease.

The author or publisher is not responsible for the use or safety of any diet, procedure or treatment mentioned in this book. The author or publisher is not responsible for errors or omissions that may exist.

Warning

The Book is for informational purposes only and before taking on any diet, treatment or medical procedure, it is recommended to consult with your primary health care provider.

Our books are available at

1. Amazon.com
2. Barnes and Noble
3. Itunes
4. Kobo
5. Smashwords
6. Google Play Books

Table of Contents

Introduction

Did you know that more and more of us are getting obsessed with our weights, in the twenty first century? That is because the demands of society and the dictates of fashion have deemed it necessary for us to be as thin as telegraph poles in order to be considered attractive.

This sort of obsession has appeared only in the twentieth century, after the First World War, when there was a dearth of food to eat, and half of the world was starving. It was then that the androgynous look was born, especially in matters of fashion, and people who were totally skeletal in form and figure were considered to be cool, hep, and "with it."

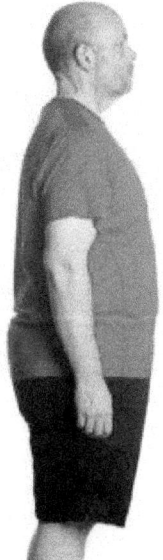 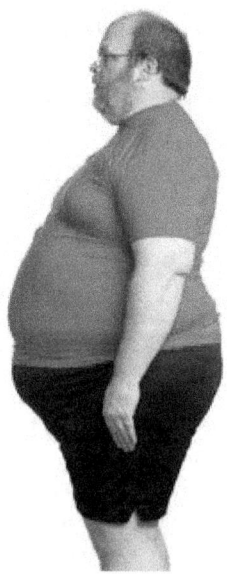

Time has gone by, the food availability situation has changed but still the notion that you need to be thin and slim with zero fat is still persisting in the mind, heart, body and soul of nearly everybody out there, who wants to be considered attractive, good-looking and desirable.

Let me give you an example. Pick up any stupid soppy romantic fiction novel out there. Look at the hero. He is musclebound with zero fat. Look at the heroine – she is slim, thin, and possibly bony. Fiction writers want us to believe that these are the only sort of people, who can be attractive to each other, and this is the subconscious notion being fed in, into us, through the media, the books we read, and any other publications out there.

This book is going to tell you all about weight watching, getting obsessed about your weight, weight charts, and everything else you need to know all about proper weight.

We know that being overweight is bad for health, because that can lead to plenty of diseases, especially cardiac problems. On the other hand, starvation is also going to lead to even more diseases, because you are now going to be suffering from malnutrition. So this book is going to tell you how to get rid of that weight watching obsession and stop being a weighing scales addict.

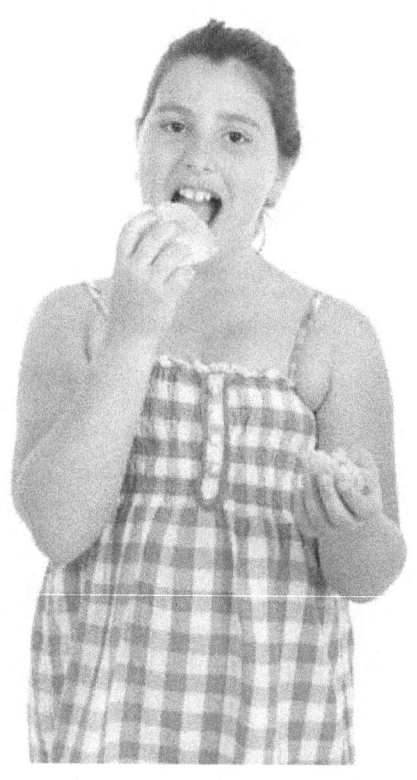

Uncontrolled eating habits during childhood itself can lead to weight problems as an adult.

Are You a Closet Weighing Scales Addict?

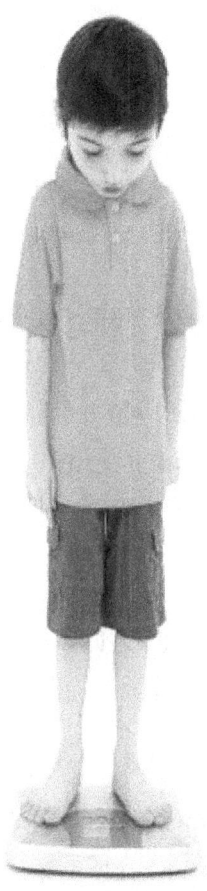

This may sound amusing to you, but believe it or not, they are a large percentage of us out there, who cannot pass a weighing scale without checking our weights. We are also obsessed by our weights, and the moment we get that information that we have put on 2 pounds, we are going to put on another 2 pounds of gloom on our minds, bodies and souls.

Oh my, oh my, I have put on 2 pounds, I have to get rid of it fast, and what am I going to do, and boy, I look so ugly,... And so on and so forth, are the thoughts which run like a demented little squirrels through our minds.

On the other hand, many of us would not go near the weighing scale, even if someone paid us to do so. That is because we are afraid of what the result is going to be. This is the outcome of our uncontrolled binging, in clear black and white. This also means that we will now have to subject ourselves to a rigorous and healthy diet in order to get back into a state of good health.

And how many of us have the self-discipline to do exactly that? Not I for sure. And that is why, when we fall sick, we find ourselves looking for shortcuts in the form of crash diets which can supposedly help us lose weight. Unfortunately, these fads and crash diets are capable of destroying any remaining vestiges of good health which we had.

Whether you are obsessed with your weight or are scared of finding out what it is, it is a fact that the presiding deity and top priority in the lives and times of many of the dieters and weight watchers out there is the ubiquitous weighing scale.

In medieval times men and women who were well-rounded were considered to be attractive, because at that time only rich people could have enough of food on their tables in order to get fat. The common people had to struggle for meals. And that is why the general populace was totally half starved. I remember a story I read about eighteenth and nineteenth century Cornwall, where the girls of the village were extremely beautiful. That was because they did not have enough of food to eat! So with a hard life and just limited food to eat, they had managed to turn out to be slim and well-shaped goddesses.

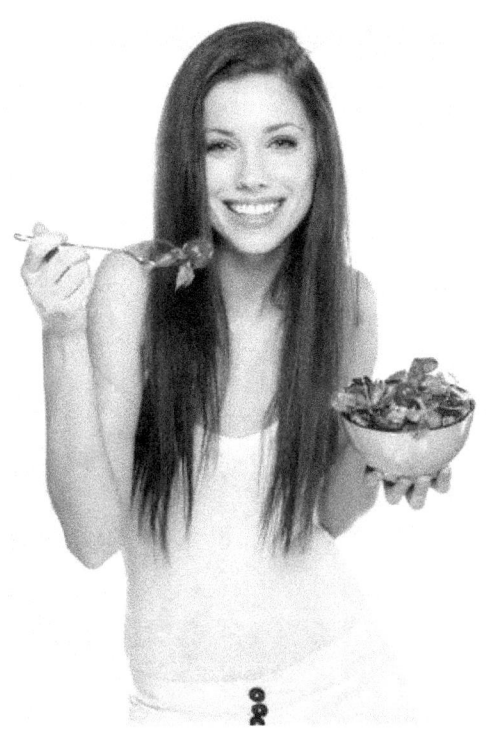

If you really want to diet, it is better you eat something which comes in the healthy food category.

On the other hand, it being a male oriented society, the amount of which was available was given to the boys of the family because they were supposed to go out fishing in the sea and they needed all the nutrition and nourishment they could get.

Some of these boys definitely were not so willing to work, but they were always willing to eat. And so they grew an attractive, pudgy and porcine like.

As technological development got more and more advanced all over the world, and the passing of time provided lots of food available to everybody, is it a wonder that the first priority of those generations was to eat and eat and eat.

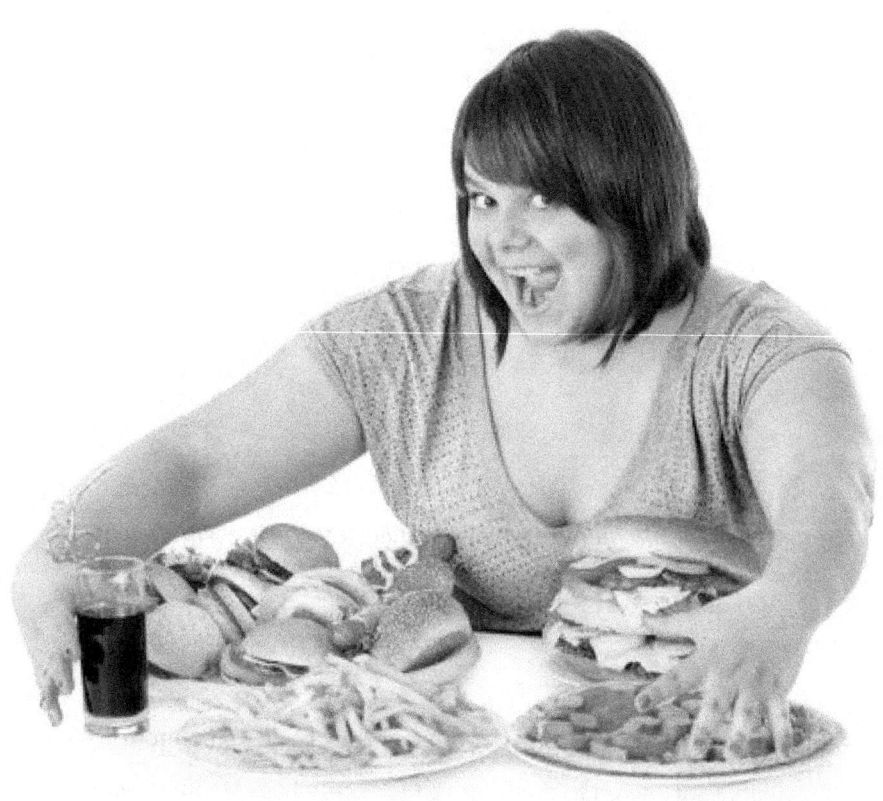

Food glorious food!

What a wonder it was to have enough of food so that they could grow well covered. But then they found that too much of food and too little of exercise meant stodgy, unshapely, and unattractive bodies. And so the idea of dieting began, but only as a fad in the initial stages.

It is a well-known fact that one of the greatest poseurs of Regency England managed to keep himself in the limelight by requesting just vinegar and biscuits for dinner at every party he graced. He was supposedly on a diet. Nobody bothered to check up what Lord Byron had, when he came back home, as hungry as a wolf. He dined off partridges, and puddings, beef and burgundy, soup and soufflés, so one would not be surprised to note that he did not lose an ounce of weight.

However, today, we are so socially conscious that if we go out to parties, nearly everybody is dieting, and is going to nibble just zero fat sandwiches, low-calorie salads and other diet conscious food items while bemoaning the fact that they have put on this itsy-bitsy amount of weight.

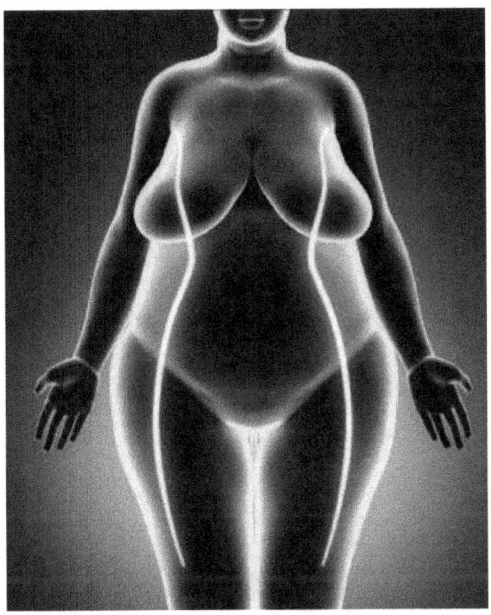

Earlier, women were more conscious about their looks and their weight, but nowadays, one is noticing that men have also become very looks and weight conscious. About 80 years ago, a well covered man would be considered to be a macho/prosperous man, who was earning well. He had enough to eat. Today, his great-grandson is looking for the easiest diet with which he can get rid of that extra fat which he put on, sitting in front of the TV or the computer.

What is the weight that these obsessively motivated people aspire to reach? The truth is that most of them would like their weights to keep falling, but they would be ready to settle to a figure given as "ideal". This ideal figure has come down as the perfect figure for a person of their height at the height weight charts one normally in every doctor's clinic.

Weight Reducing Clinics

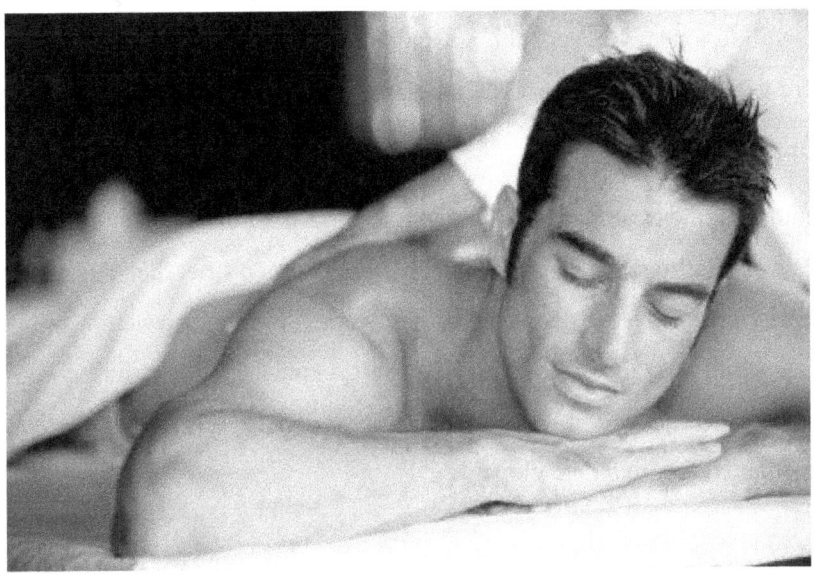

Weight reducing clinics have a number of programs which supposedly help you reduce weight. These include aromatic oil massages and fat burning therapies.

Cashing in on this obsession, there are plenty of weight reduction clinics which have sprouted up overnight, and are doing big business. These clinics advertise intensively with before and after photographs, of people who they claim have been patients at their clinic. These people have lost an unbelievable amount of weight through their programs, according to the advertisements.

Are such advertisements really true?

Well, I can just say that in some cases, they are true, because one of the success stories was my uncle. He was about 40 pounds overweight! And he was still less than 40 years old. So somebody told him to get into one of the more expensive and supposedly popular weight reducing clinics, in the city. He did.

He under grew treatment for about two years, and of course the monthly fees was exorbitant. Along with that, he was put on a strict diet, and a strict exercise regime by the people who were helping him to lose weight. When we saw him at a cousin's wedding, we were astonished at his trim figure, and of course his youthful good looks. We were definitely very impressed with that weight reducing clinic.

The only problem was that uncle could not manage to eat anything at the wedding, because he was not allowed to do so. That was to make sure that his weight kept constant because according to him, he was prone to gaining weight. This is what the professionals in the clinic had told him.

So use some common sense. Exercise on your own for two hard years, and put yourself on a strict, steady, and sensible diet. And you are going to see yourself losing weight within six months.

By the way, uncle was one of these before and after success stories, with his photos prominently displayed in journals and in newspapers. People used to come and congratulate him for looking so good and losing so much of weight. In fact, he was paid to market the clinic by showing himself off as visible proof of their success rate! But he did not tell them about the strict diet and the tough exercise sessions which he had to undergo in that weight reducing clinic.

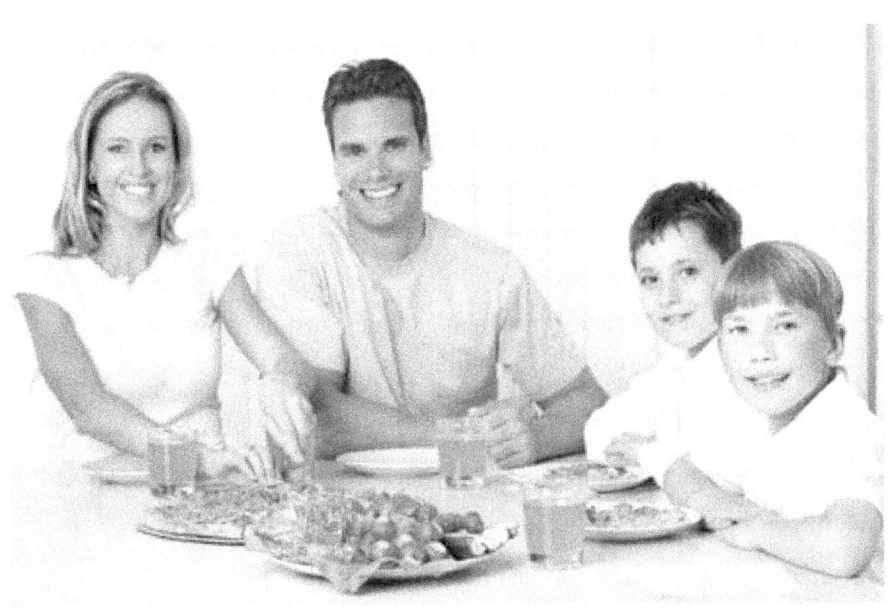

Healthy and proper regular diets mean less of worry of growing obese.

Apart from these claims, these clinics are also reinforcing a very dangerous social message. This message is that these clinics claim that this weight loss is going make the people happier, more desirable, more self confident and even more successful!

Can you understand this covert subconscious message being fed to you? It means that if you are fat, you are definitely not happy. You do not have any self-confidence. People are not going to find you attractive. You may not get your desired job just because you are a little bit overweight. On the other hand, if you come to their clinic and join their weight reduction program right now, you are going to find yourself happier, more self-confident, more attractive, and everybody is going to want to hire you.

If you read any of these ads, you are going to notice that the clinics do not give any details of the treatments they offer. However, they are going to hint at esoteric treatments over which they have a monopoly. These are secret treatments, over which only their own professionals have mastery and command.

I went into one of these weight reducing clinics, just to interview their owner about two decades ago when I was a subeditor for one of the most well-known magazines in our country. At that time, weight reducing clinics had just begun to come into existence in the area. The inside of the clinic was full of a gym, a hot sauna bath, a massage parlor, a kitchen where food was being made specially for the clients, a lab where a white coated figure was mixing some things in a mortar and pestle and nothing else. And this was supposed to be a place where you were going to reduce your weight.

I happen to be naturally cynical, so I decided that this was a con game. But I was not going to tell anybody that, because once a person has decided to enroll himself into a weight reducing program, nobody can budge him. He knows what is best for himself. He is going to put himself in the hands of possible charlatans.

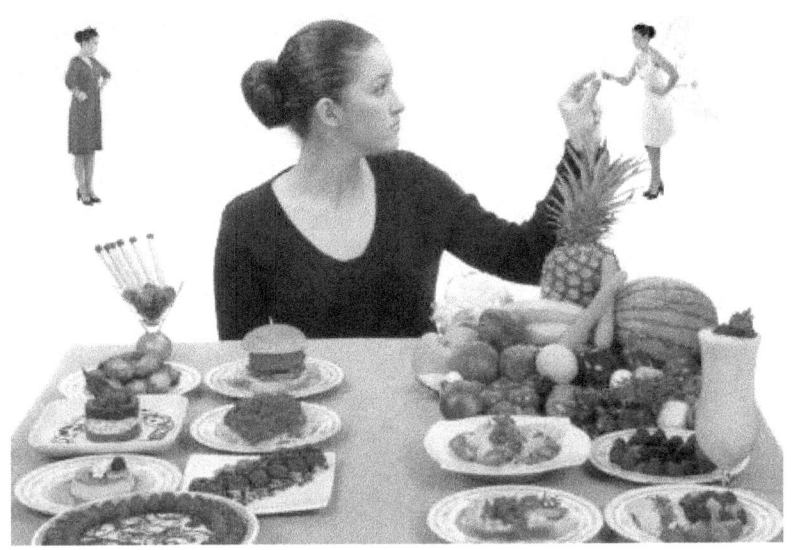

Eat this. Do not eat that.

When one is taken in by these ads and joins their programs, one is usually going to find that one is and powders, pills, and potions that are touted as being able to destroy the appetite, even as they provide essential nutrition. Also, these people are going to be given a diet chart to which they have to adhere strictly.

Now we being humans are definitely not going to listen to anybody ordering us to do something. Even if it is for our own good. That is why these professionals in the clinics managed to persuade their clients that if they take anything else apart from the diet chart items, the medicines which are being given to them are not going to take effect!

Notice this bit of chicanery? Just imagine that you are being given sugar and calcium powder as a weight reducing magic medicine. You are impressed by an experienced "doctor" telling you that this magic medicine has come down the ages and only his clinic knows the secret of it. But it is only going to work, when it works it is magic in tandem with the items given in the diet chart. Eat anything else and the magic is going to stop having its beneficial effect.

Oh my, you tell yourself, you cannot afford to do that. So you stop eating items like red meat, bread, biscuits, and other items, which are going to cause a weight gain. And you stick to your diet chart. No wonder, you are going to lose weight! And you think it was because of that magic sugar and calcium powder which was given to you in small packets at that clinic!

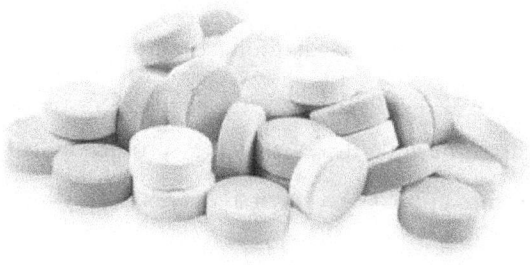

Let me tell you the truth about some of these potions and pills. In 1960, some of these weight reducing pills became very popular, because they supposedly reduced the appetites. The people who marketed them became multimillionaires overnight. Till one fine day, complaints began coming in that people who took these pills began to feel nauseated even though they had lost weight within three months of taking these pills regularly.

Those pills were opened up by the health authorities. And they were shocked to find that they were full of tapeworm eggs. This does sound nauseating, but the idea of these pill pushers was that tapeworms were parasites, and they would go into the stomach, and eat the food there. That they would also weaken the body due to their presence was one thing they definitely did not want to tell the public.

So if people are so credible and gullible, that they can eat or drink something which supposedly is going to help them reduce weight, but which actually is going to be harming their bodies long-term, well, it is their outlook.

Besides this, the clinics also offer treatments which supposedly burn away fat. These include pressure wraps which push in the fat. They are also going to extol surgical procedures like liposuction, which is going to remove the fat from your thighs, waist, and other parts of the body where the fat has accumulated.

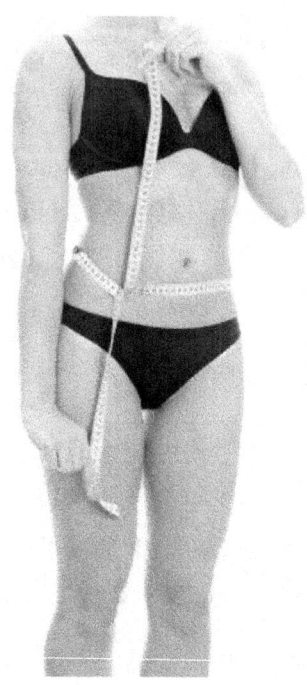

Also, there are clinics, where you are going to be told that they can staple or sew the stomach so that it can hold less food!

Anybody interfering with the natural construction of the body is definitely putting your life into jeopardy. So why do people go to these health clinics?

Driven to Look Good

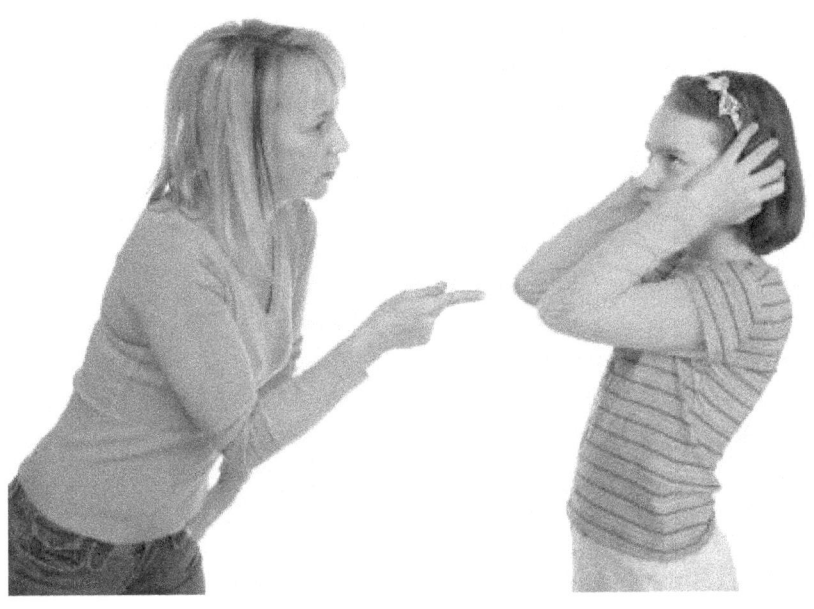

Why cannot you look like your friend Kathryn? She is smart, she is pretty, and her mama is so proud of her...

In this case, even if the younger girl is not overweight, she is being driven to look good with an odious comparison to a neighbor's child.

Being overweight is naturally bad for health, but the majority of the people who go to these clinics do not do so for health reasons. They go because they want to look good. That is because society has impressed upon their minds and psyches, that just because they are a bit overweight, they are definitely not attractive or desirable. And also they are driven there by the numbers shown on their weight scale.

This brings us to the question of how much we should really weigh. Most of us look At a height weight chart and decide what our optimum weight should be. So do the doctors. That is how they tell us that we are a certain number of pounds overweight. Sometimes they are also going to measure the amount of fat in our bodies with a machine and tell us how much fat we have, and whether it is too much! But ultimately the doctors are always going to come back to the optimum weight concept.

Optimum Weight Concept

This is supposedly a magic number which is going to get stuck in our heads. Our life is now going to be ruled by this number, and we are going to upset about it. As a result, we are also going to believe that the achievement of this number is going to make us attractive, healthy and happy. The moment we achieve it, we have conquered the world. This is going to become our goal and it is on our minds every time we take our weight.

The number on the display panel is a few pounds over that weight. And that is why we feel that our appetites are out of control. We also have the subconscious feeling that we are not in control of our lives. We could not manage to control our weight. What has happened to our self discipline?

Our weight is a few pounds above that magic number? Our self-confident dwindles away. On the other hand, it is a few pounds below that magic number. Our self-confidence has immediately been given a boost. And in this case, we are going to tell ourselves that we can eat freely now and, for at least some time, without worrying about our weights!

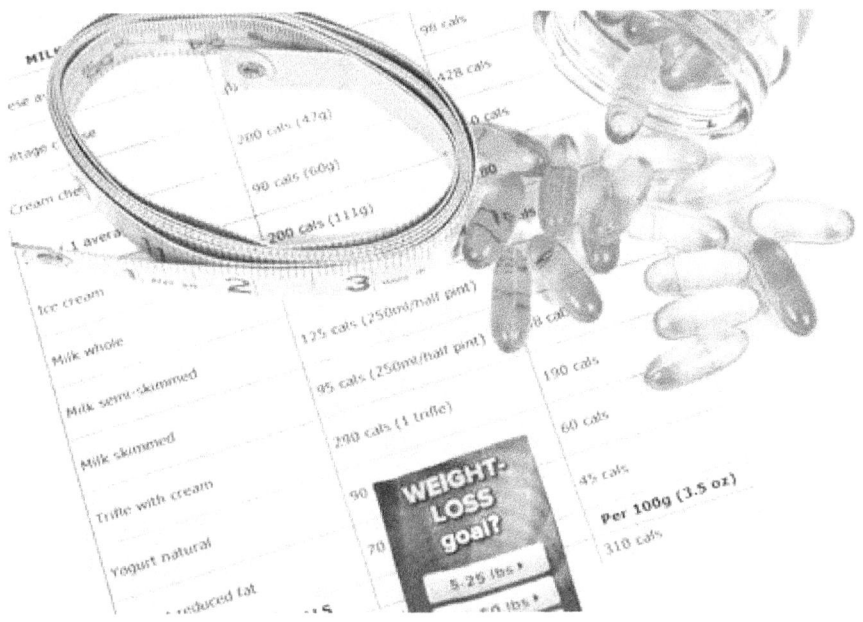

Are Weight Charts Right?

One really does not know how and when somebody decided that one weight would be the perfect poundage for a person of such and such height. Were they created by doctors on the basis of medical research? Nope. Also, the answer to this question of whether the weight charts are right is a big negative. The truth is that these height and weight charts were together in the 1950s by an American life insurance company!

When the Metropolitan Life Insurance Company decided to pep up its life insurance sales, it had to think up a new gimmick. The company just asked the policyholders to give them their heights and weights. After that they correlated them gender wise with the ages at which these people died.

From this evidence, they made up a table, of the weights at which people of different heights lived the longest! So this is how the ideal weights for different heights or either sex were thought up. They were ideal only in the sense that statistically, in the limited experience of an insurance company, people with these weights happen to live the longest during the period of time for which the study was conducted. Can anybody find any sort of logic behind this bit of marketing?

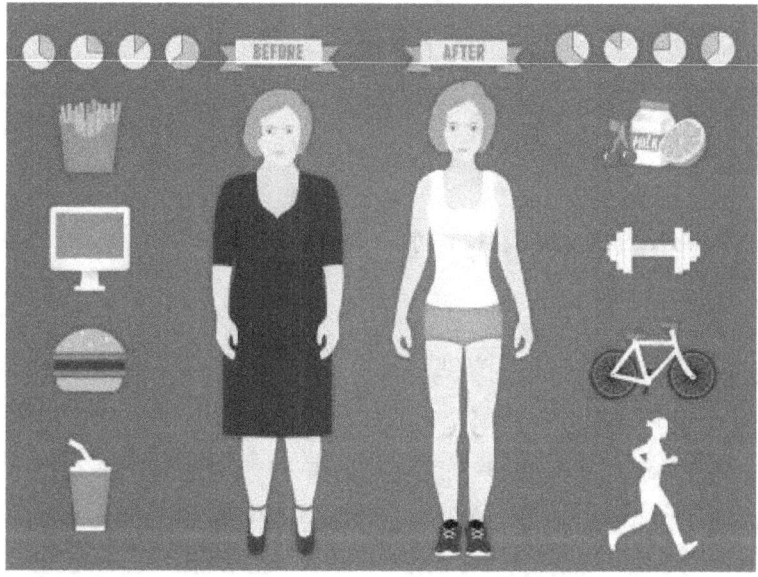

Nevertheless, these weight charts were considered to be gospel truth and even today, we are consulting these weight charts thought up an insurance company without any medical basis or background, as the ideal source of magic weights which are going to give us longevity, when they are achieved.

Remember that these charts were not created with the intention of telling people what weight they should. They were just created for a commercial insurance company so that the company could predict the probable lifespan of a client. This assessment would be done beforehand, so that the company did not have to pay out insurance money to the client's heirs after his death.

Also it was to determine the premium that he or she should pay, because he was either a "good bet" because he was not overweight and thus was possibly not prone to medical problems caused through obesity. Or he was a "bad bet", because he was so many pounds overweight and the chances of his dropping down dead, one fine morning, was thus probable and possible.

However, even today more than 60 years after the charts were tabulated, people still consider these charts to be their guide about ideal weight.

Psychological Effect of Weight Chart Watching

Remember that whenever you look at the weight chart, you are looking at something which has no medical basis but it has been in use for more than 60 years, as the Guru of ideal weight magic numbers.

If you begin to get obsessed with a piece of paper with some numbers written on it, which have absolutely no valid justification, you are putting yourself through a psychological trauma which could have been avoided if you never referred to that useless chart before!

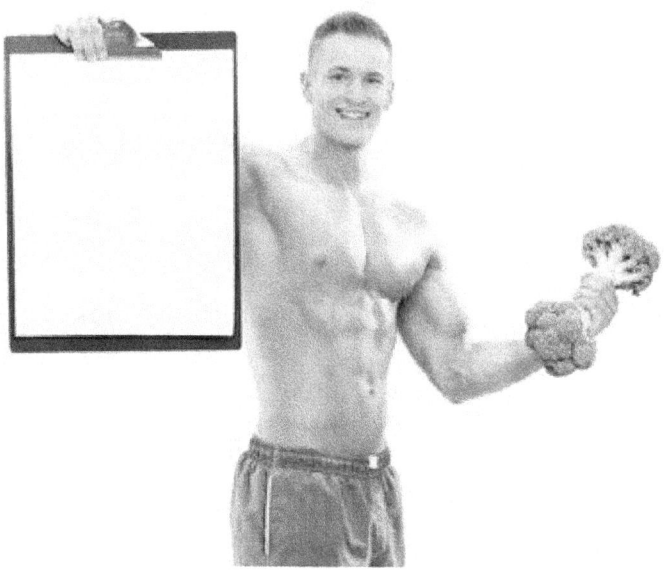

Let me give you my example.

A couple of years ago, I looked at one of these charts, because at that time I was under the impression that these had been made by experienced dietitians and doctors. And I was under the impression that they knew what they were doing when they made up these charts, based on their research and experience.

So height – 6 feet, female, my ideal weight should be 138 – 176 pounds according to the weight charts. I was seven pounds overweight. Believe it or not, I who am a normally sensible, sober, and well-balanced person, went into a flat tizzy. This had never happened before, because basically, I was underweight throughout my life. I immediately did something I had never done before.

I went on a diet. It was a crash diet. I intended to get those 7 pounds off within the next 15 days. Now, for all those people were out there, and who enjoy dieting, let me tell you that this is the most harmful thing that you could do to a body which is used to regular nourishment and plenty of nutrients, three times a day.

A diet means that you are starving your body of essential nutrients which it needs to keep itself functioning properly. Consciously going on a diet, when you are healthy, but you want to lose some weight is one of the most foolish things which a normal person could do. Sometimes doctors recommend diet for people who are ill, so that they can lose weight, which is potentially life-threatening.

But here you are, a healthy person, with just this little bit of weight on you, and you decide to starve yourself. So that is what I did. I went on the Israeli army diet, told to me by one of my Israeli army friends. They normally do this diet to keep to the required weight of 72 kg. I do not know about the psychological reason for that particular magic number which is considered to be healthy for a person who maybe 5 foot nine or may be 6 foot two, but both of these have to be 72 kg to be considered healthy soldiers by their Army doctors!

Anyway, the first two days I just had apples and nothing else. The next two days I had boiled chicken and nothing else. The last two days I had as much ease as I could eat and nothing else.

Believe me, on the seventh day I had lost 4 pounds. But the problem was that this unusual diet had such a detrimental effect on my psyche, and on my mood, that it took me three months to get back to normal. And it took me one year to get back to my normal weight which was *7 pounds overweight.*

This was what my body preferred and this kept me functioning properly, happily and in a healthy fashion. But if I had gone by the charts, I would be 7 pounds underweight in order to achieve that magic figure.

I would not be healthy, I would not be in a good mood, because I had starved myself and also, the body would need to adjust itself to a sudden weight loss. This would cause the sagging of muscles as well as tissue.

Think about that.

When I lost that weight, it showed up immediately on my face. I had gone on that crash diet because I had to attend a wedding. According to me, I was looking good, because I did not look fat and plump. According to the guests, friends, acquaintances and relatives, they were worried because my face looked haggard. Was not I eating properly? Was I sick or something? What had I done to myself? My face looked all skull and bones.

I did not enjoy that wedding at all.

However, finally, some doctors put their heads and brains together, and decided that these weight charts were quackery and gimmicks, but there should be some scientific basis for calculating the ideal weight.

And so the body mass index came into existence.

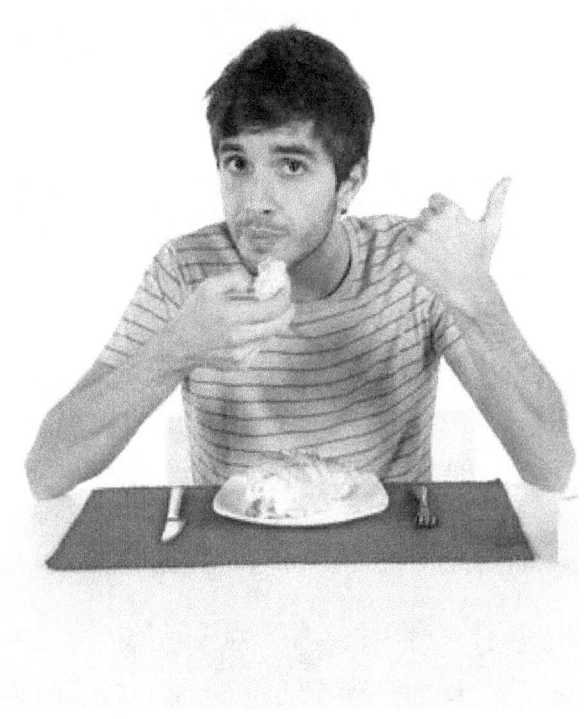

Body Mass Index – BMI

The calculation of body mass index also uses the parameters of height and weight, to tell you whether you are underweight or overweight. Ultimately with the body mass index, you are going to come down to ideal weights which are going to fall within a certain range.

The Body Mass Index is an 19th-century equation which was first worked out by a mathematician called Lambert Adolphe Jacques Quetelet. The insurance company employees making weight charts in the 1960s definitely did not take this mathematical calculation into account.

According to him, BMI is equal to the weight in kilograms/pounds divided by the height in meters squared.

So if you have a BMI of under 20 means that you are underweight. If you have a BMI of 20 – 25, that means you are just right and if it is between 26 and 30, it means that you are underweight. A BMI of 31 – 40 means that you are frankly obese.

The BMI is going to measure fat mass accurately, speedily and specifically. Even so, it basically comes down to the two factors of weight and height. However, the range is going to give you the chance to factor in matters of frame and size, but the emphasis is still going to be on your weight.

Nevertheless, nowadays, fitness experts and doctors have a different take on your general health. They are looking beyond the weighing machine. The number game is getting to be obsolete in medical circles, even though it is so popular among many individuals obsessed with their weights.

Research has shown that there are many other factors and indicators beside weight, which have to be taken into consideration in determining whether a person is in danger of developing weight related problems. In fact, using just the pound count as a measure of health and fitness can be inaccurate as well as misleading.

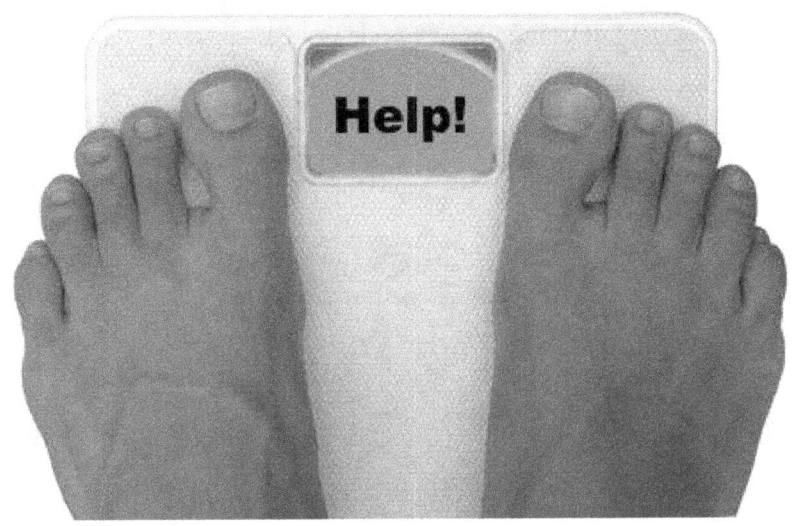

In fact, I would add my own bit to these factors. Scientists have not researched on genetic background as a contributing factor to ailments which are basically weight related. Also remember that underweight people are possibly going to have more body fat than others who look bulkier and heavier. This can depend on their body type and their genetic background.

Also, people who are underweight may be prone to high blood pressure and they are not going to suspect it because they are under the impression that high blood pressure is an ailment common to people who are suffering from obesity or overweight problems.

Thus, even underweight people are going to be most likely candidates for heart attacks, when compared with overweight people. The people who are overweight are more likely to be watchful about what they eat and about taking exercise. But a person was underweight is going to consider himself healthy, because according to him, there is no question of his suffering from heart ailments. So he may not exercise, and he is going to eat whatever he wants without any hold. And naturally, such carelessness is going to lead to health problems later in life.

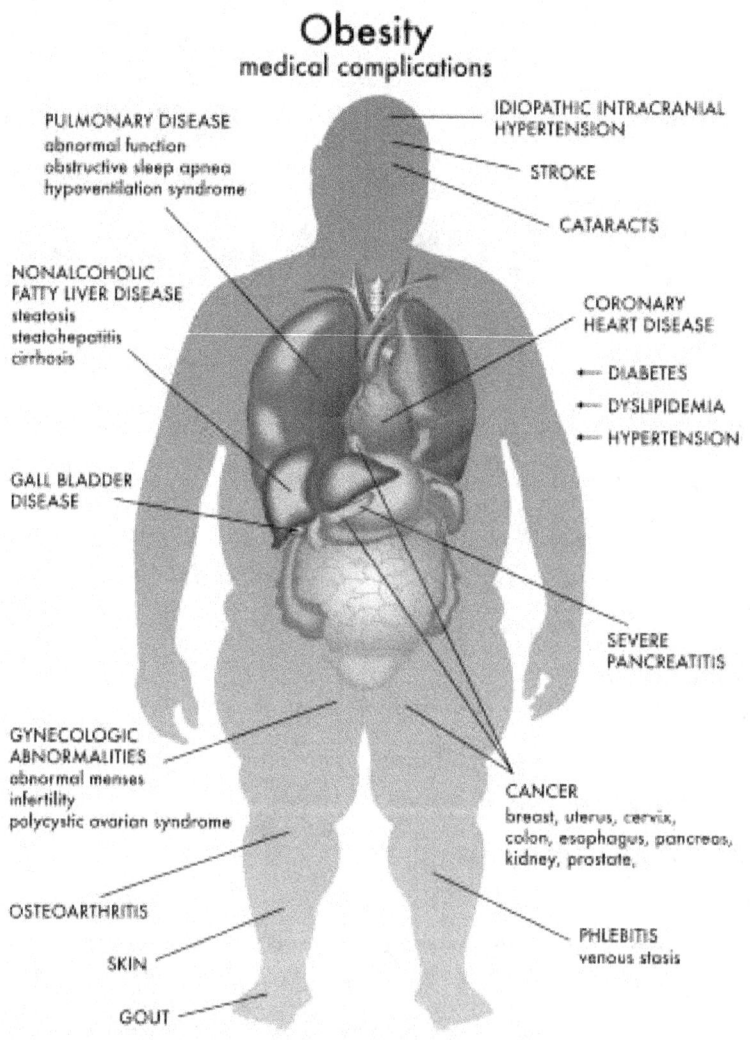

Obesity
medical complications

PULMONARY DISEASE
abnormal function
obstructive sleep apnea
hypoventilation syndrome

IDIOPATHIC INTRACRANIAL
HYPERTENSION

STROKE

CATARACTS

NONALCOHOLIC
FATTY LIVER DISEASE
steatosis
steatohepatitis
cirrhosis

CORONARY
HEART DISEASE

DIABETES

DYSLIPIDEMIA

HYPERTENSION

GALL BLADDER
DISEASE

SEVERE
PANCREATITIS

GYNECOLOGIC
ABNORMALITIES
abnormal menses
infertility
polycystic ovarian syndrome

CANCER
breast, uterus, cervix,
colon, esophagus, pancreas,
kidney, prostate,

OSTEOARTHRITIS

PHLEBITIS
venous stasis

SKIN

GOUT

Health risk of Slim People

People can be slim and still be unhealthy for various reasons. I am giving you my example. I was genetically programmed to be slim, because I inherited slim genes from my paternal ancestors. However, that was definitely no indication of good health. I definitely was not healthy throughout my life until I began to put on a little bit of weight. That gave my body bulk, and also I began taking enough of nutrition in order to strengthen my immunity system, with an increase in my diet.

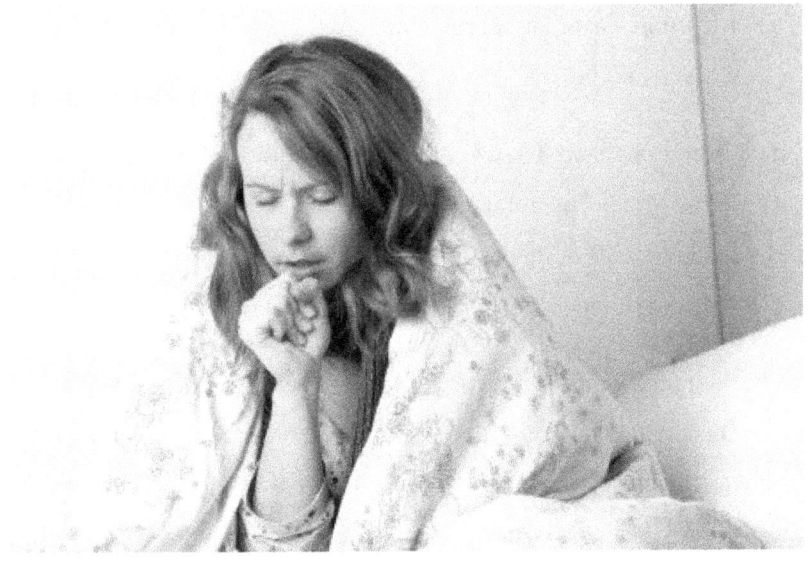

A weak immunity system may make you more vulnerable to infections and diseases.

Also, many people may find their weight is low, because they do not do any exercise at all. That means their muscles are light and have not had the capacity to grow. Also, sportsmen on the other hand can have dense and heavy muscles and weight. This is due to their regular exercise regimen, which can make them look bulky and "fat", but incidentally, they are very healthy.

Let me give you an example of a 16-year-old lad of my acquaintance. Exercise was anathema to him. And because he did not exercise, his appetite was also quite low. That was because he did not feel hungry. So he was as thin as a rake and also had the personality of a thorough going goof. That was because he looked half starved and did not have the energy to show any sort of spirit, enthusiasm, or energy to do anything except with dragging feet and a lethargic, sulky mien.

And then things changed. He was selected into military college. That meant physical PT as soon as he got up at 6 o'clock for a couple of hours. Then he went in for his breakfast, then studies, then lunch, and more outdoor exercise, tea, and dinner interspersed with exercise outdoors and studies.

When he came back after three months on his first leave, all of us looked at him with our mouths open. In fact, in the opinion of everybody who beheld him, he was the most beautiful youngster they had ever seen, with the glow of health on his face, and with rippling muscles. And there was no question of his being underweight or overweight. Military college was really wonderful!

His tread was confident and he had also acquired an attitude. This attitude is still present three decades later, today, even though those muscles have turned into flab because for him, exercise is such a bore, and he could not be bothered to walk, when he has vehicles at his command! This is what sedentary lifestyles do to you.

Other Factors Affecting Good Health

Naturally, none of us have the willpower to put ourselves under military college, in order to become healthy. Also, both the scales and the BMI may fail to account for weight from muscle and therefore, a lean and fit athlete may be put into the overweight or even obese category. In the same manner, any elderly person may appear to have a good BMI, but may have high levels of body fat because of the low muscle mass.

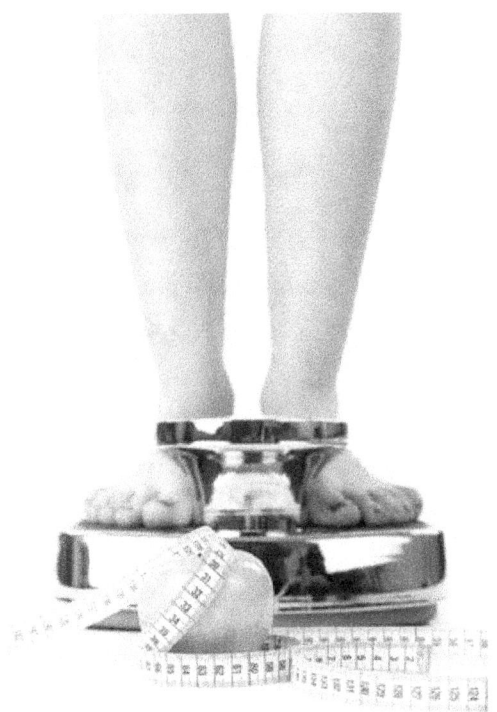

In the same manner, smokers are also going to have low weight. That is because smoking tends to keep the weight down. One reason it does is because the tobacco is capable of killing all that appetite which was ravenous when you were not smoking. So because you would rather stick a coffee nail in your mouth than eat something healthy, naturally, you are going to have a low weight. Also, people were suffering from depression are not going to have overweight problems because they do not want to eat anything at all. In fact, they may suffer from malnutrition and starvation.

So if a person is suffering from depression and is also a heavy smoker, and underweight, you can definitely not call him healthy.

Again, if you are comparing three people who wear the same and are about the same height, they may not be equally healthy or unhealthy. One may have heavy muscles. The other one may have plenty of flab. The third may be a bit overweight due to water retention.

Also, these three individuals are going to have totally different levels of and durance, aerobic capacity, flexibility, blood pressure, stamina, muscle tone, cholesterol and blood sugar. These levels are definitely more important than just their weights in determining their health status.

According to health researchers, the circumference of the waste, and not just the amount of extra fat there is so important that it should be taken into consideration together with such risk factors as blood sugar levels, high blood pressure, genetic probability of heart disease, smoking and the lack of exercise, when evaluating a person's general health.

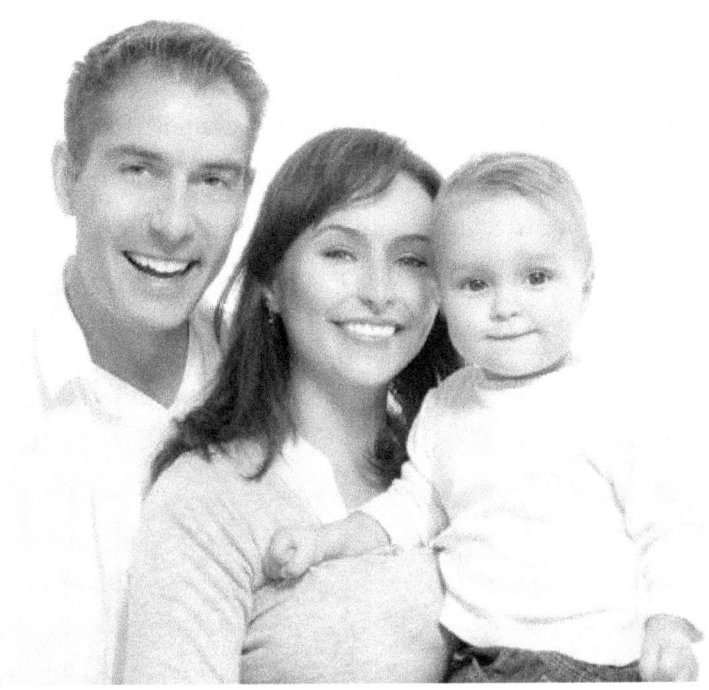

Healthy and happy!

Dos and Don'ts While Weight Watching

If you are young or if you are very conscious about your looks, remember not to take your weight after you have done a workout or you have undergone a sauna bath. The scales are going to show less than your actual weight at these times that is because of water loss.

Do not take your weight the morning after you have had alcoholic drinks at a party the night before. Also, if you have drunk a lot of coffee, this is also going to affect your weight. Both of these food items have a dehydrating effect and that is why the weight, which is going to show on the scales is going to be lower than your actual weight.

Also, if you are a weighing scale addict, do not take your weight after a heavy meal. I have seen people doing that because their consciences are pricking them. That food still has to be digested, assimilated and eliminated. But you have just had some heavy meals and you are wondering whether it has any effect on your weight. And if you find the scales moving clockwise, you are going to be steeped in guilt, and gloom.

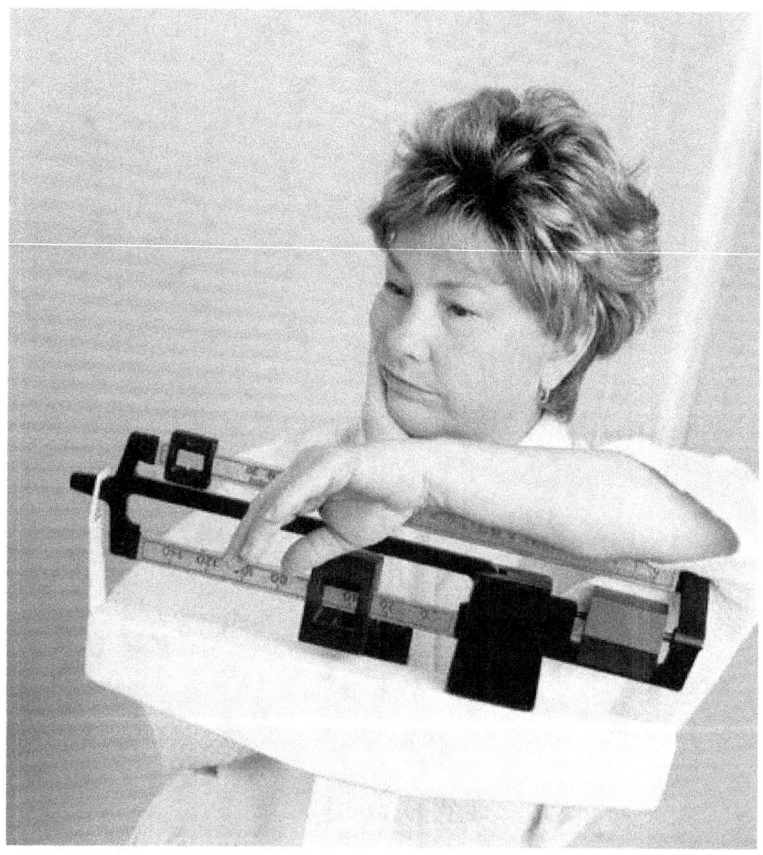

Also, women should not weigh themselves during their premenstrual week. This is when water retention is the highest and it is also why you feel bloated. And this is the reason why so many women get depressed before their periods, because they think that they have grown fat. Remember that this is water retention only, which is going to be eliminated within the week.

And above all, do not be like the lady in the picture on the previous page. Weight loss is done slowly and steadily and definitely not overnight.

Eating Habit Disorders

I was surprised to learn that even young men have begun suffering from eating habit disorders because these eating disorders among young women were considered to be very common during the last 30 – 40 years. However, in the last 10 years, young men have also begun falling victims to anorexia and bulimia.

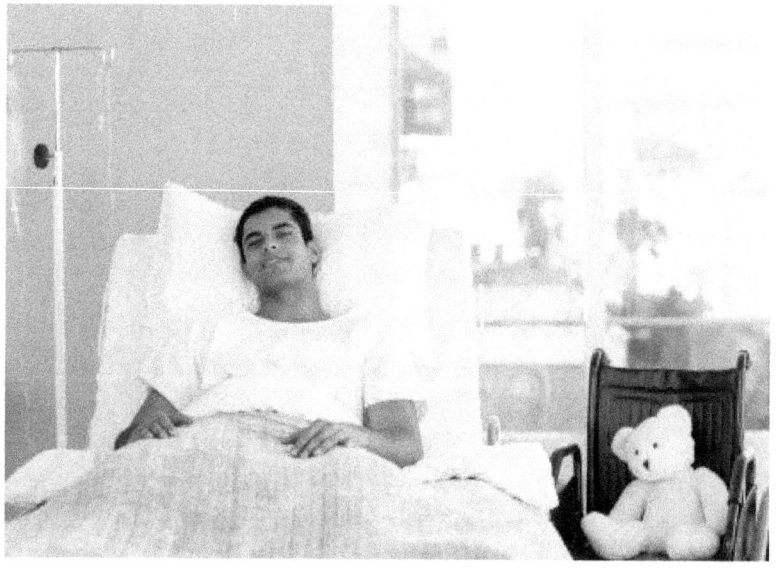

Starvation and malnutrition can be potentially life-threatening.

Young women have been dealing with these problems for decades, especially when they stop eating in order to look slim and thin. That is because they have been bombarded with media versions of body images which are almost unrealistic.

And then some foolish starlet gets lots of publicity, because she has gone on to a crash diet and now has a zero fat body. The media touts her to be extremely beautiful and desirable. What they do not know is that this foolish woman has completely ruined her health, and it is going to take her anywhere between 5 to 7 years to become healthy again.

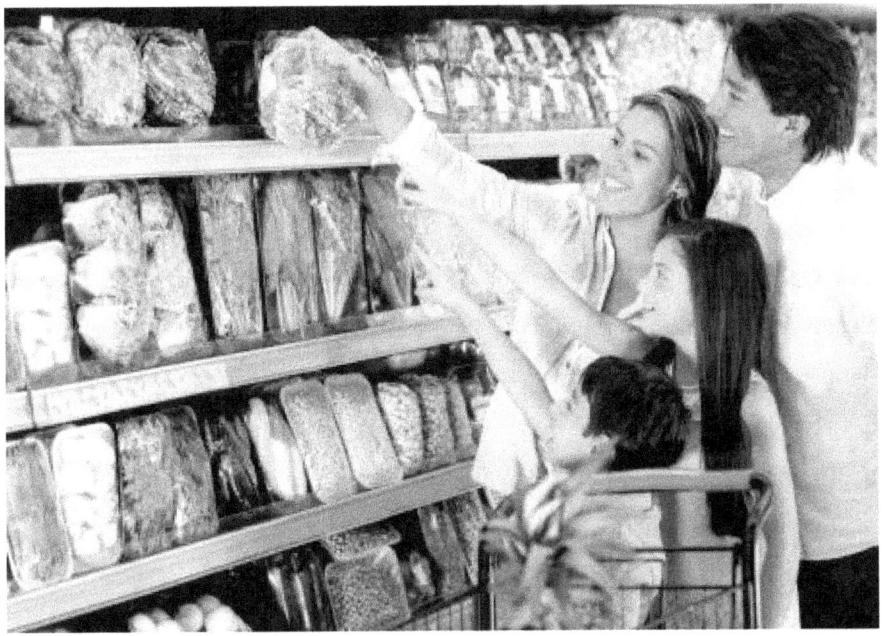

A healthy diet means avoiding eating disorders.

That is because the body needs a little bit of fat in order to keep functioning properly. She has now made herself vulnerable to diseases because her diet has deprived her of essential nutrients which were necessary to keep her healthy and her body functioning properly.

About 10% of the young people suffering from eating disorders in the world today are men. We may not believe that, but there has been a disturbing trend in the rise of fitness freaks who desperately want to look like the figures of cover men on health magazines.

That is why they have also begun to take steroids in order to get that sixpack or eight pack. Look on any fiction book cover. The hero – even if he is a psychological and mental mess – is going to have a body of a bodybuilder or weight lifter. Those overtly bulging muscles are supposed to be masculine, attractive, and desirable.

These young men who suffer from eating disorders need counseling in order to survive. Remember that not all dieters are going to fall victim to dangerous eating disorders as anorexia nervosa and bulimia. Nevertheless, dissatisfaction with your own body and an obsession with losing weight and continuous dieting can make you enjoy life much less. It is also going to make you less productive and less successful because you are obsessed with one top priority – losing weight.

Conclusion

Rather than aiming at a so-called ideal weight, you should make sure that your levels of cholesterol, blood sugar, triglycerides and blood pressure falls within the normal range is you should also be so active, so that your heart rate and lung capacity remains healthy. Also, you need to aim to have strong muscles and flexible bodies.

Weight is a very emotive issue which can cause eating disorders like anorexia and bulimia. Princess Di suffered from it, because she was so much in the public eye. Your young teenager may be suffering from it, because she thinks her puppy fat makes her look unattractive. And that is why she stops eating properly. Or she may stop eating altogether.

Overweight people may have a low self-esteem and they think that they are failures because they are unable to meet the societal expectation of all women should be slim and beautiful and also all men should have bodies like WWF wrestlers or models.

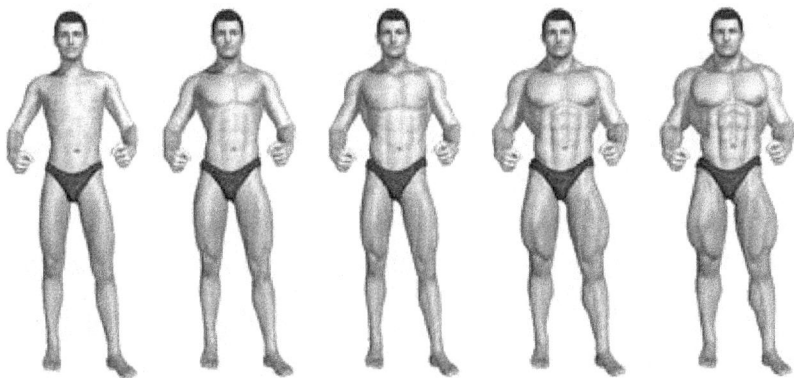

Consider all this to be social fiddle faddle .

This social pressure, and sometimes other problems in their personal lives may give rise to eating disorders and depression.

So if you find somebody in your vicinity, especially a teenager eating minuscule quantities of food, or skipping meals when you are not around, make sure that he is not suffering from eating disorders. The result of this is going to be that he is going to start losing weight and begin to look listless and pale.

Such people may say that they are overweight, even when you see them wasting away visibly. There have been cases when such people waste away so much that even drips in hospitals cannot keep them alive. They have literally died of starvation. And the reason why they have brought this upon themselves is because of societal pressure to look good. According to them looking good means being slim. But when you talk to a psychoanalyst, he is going to tell you that your eating disorder is because of low self-esteem.

Some of these people may control their eating for some time, and then go into binges. This is anorexia bulimia. And afterwards, they are going to purge themselves of the food which they have eaten before giving it a chance to assimilate in their bodies.

People suffering from such a disorder may not have a clear concept of what they look like that is why they intend to starve themselves.

Many people think that they are behaving in this manner because of a deep desire to lose weight and become slim. However, this is also a psychological problem. There might be some underlying cause for this, like perhaps the person considers himself unloved or blames himself for something which is beyond his control.

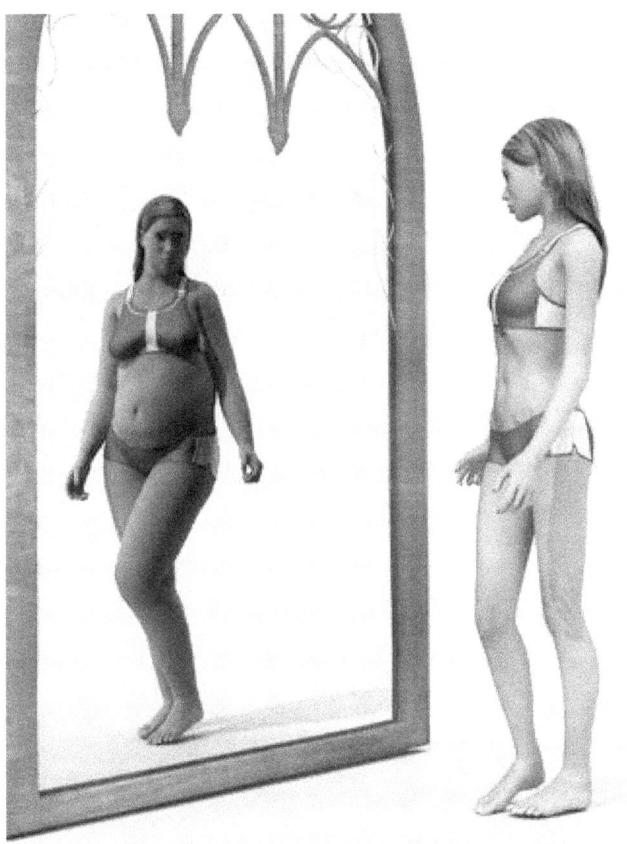

This old guilt or self blame, along with the precious society puts on young people, expecting them to look attractive and beautiful all the time may cause them to become bulimic. They are going to try not to eat, but when the demands of their body cannot be resisted, they are going to eat in an uncontrolled manner. After that guilt is going to make them purge their meals.

This behavioral pattern is very dangerous. It is going to cause damage to the food pipe. Also, some patients have literally been known to starve themselves to death. Just because they were not given counseling and proper treatment at the right time.

Make no mistake about it. Being overweight is that for health and we are all going to look better when we do not have the beer barrels, heavy hips, triple chins and thunder thighs. But that does not mean that you begin to obsess with your weight.

I hope this book has given you plenty of information on how you can stop yourself from harming yourself with dieting, unless recommended by the doctor and obsessive weight watching.

Live Long, Live Healthy and Prosper!

Author Bio

Dueep Jyot Singh is a Management and IT Professional who managed to gather Postgraduate qualifications in Management and English and Degrees in Science, French and Education while pursuing different enjoyable career options like being an hospital administrator, IT,SEO and HRD Database Manager/ trainer, movie , radio and TV scriptwriter, theatre artiste and public speaker, lecturer in French, Marketing and Advertising, ex-Editor of Hearts On Fire (now known as Solstice) Books Missouri USA, advice columnist and cartoonist, publisher and Aviation School trainer, ex-moderator on Medico.in, banker, student councilor ,travelogue writer … among other things!

One fine morning, she decided that she had enough of killing herself by Degrees and went back to her first love -- writing. It's more enjoyable! She already has 48 published academic and 14 fiction- in- different- genre books under her belt.

When she is not designing websites or making Graphic design illustrations for clients , she is browsing through old bookshops hunting for treasures, of which she has an enviable collection – including R.L. Stevenson, O.Henry, Dornford Yates, Maurice Walsh, De Maupassant, Victor Hugo, Sapper, C.N. Williamson, "Bartimeus" and the crown of her collection- Dickens "The Old Curiosity Shop," and "Martin Chuzzlewit" and so on… Just call her "Renaissance Woman") - collecting herbal remedies, acting like Universal Helping Hand/Agony Aunt, or escaping to her dear mountains for a bit of exploring, collecting herbs and plants and trekking.

Check out some of the other JD-Biz Publishing books

Gardening Series on Amazon

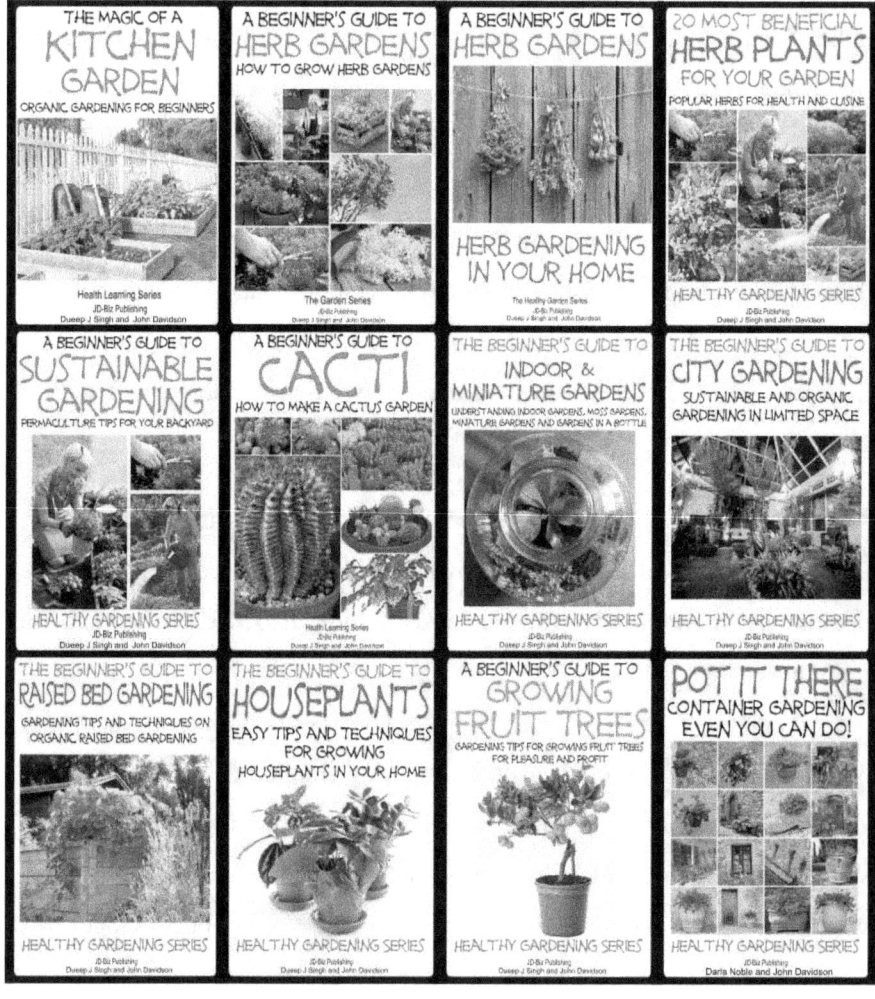

Health Learning Series

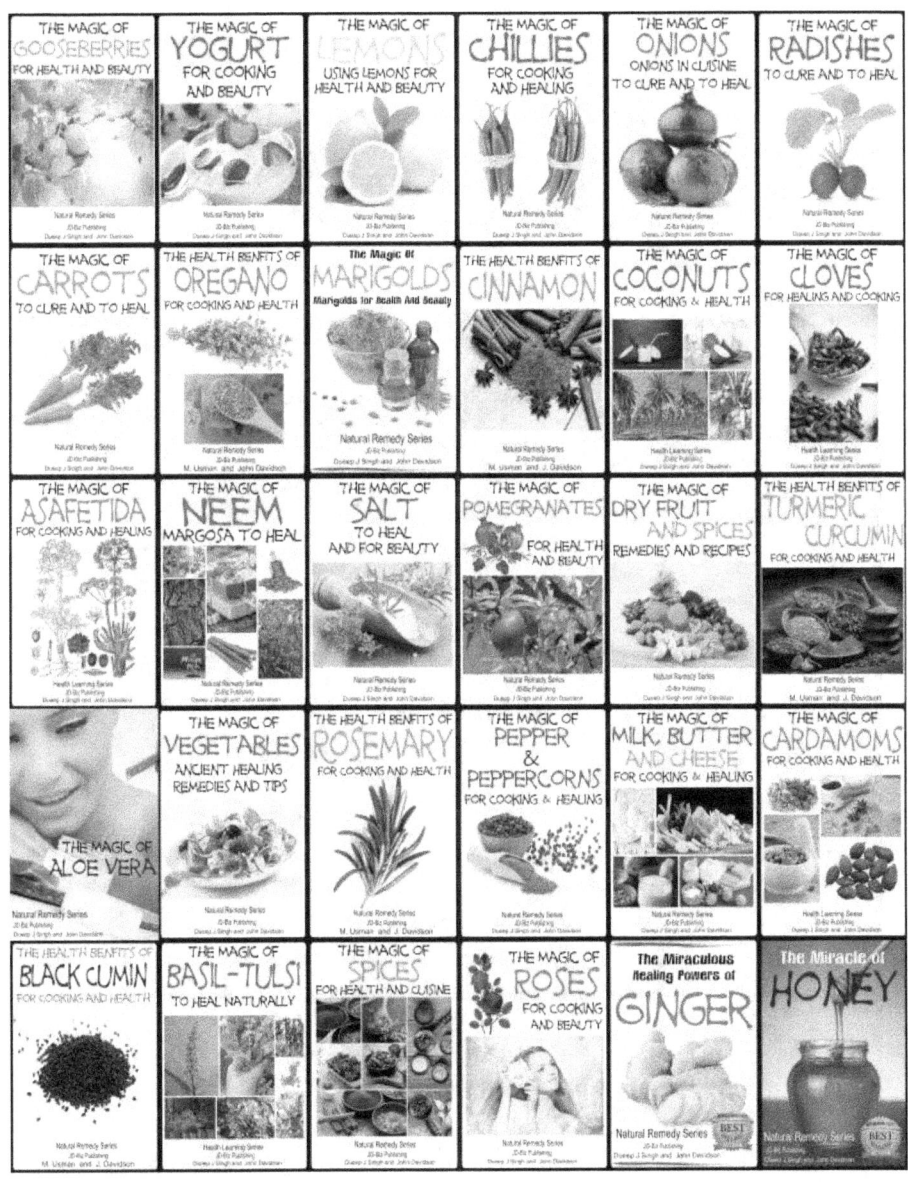

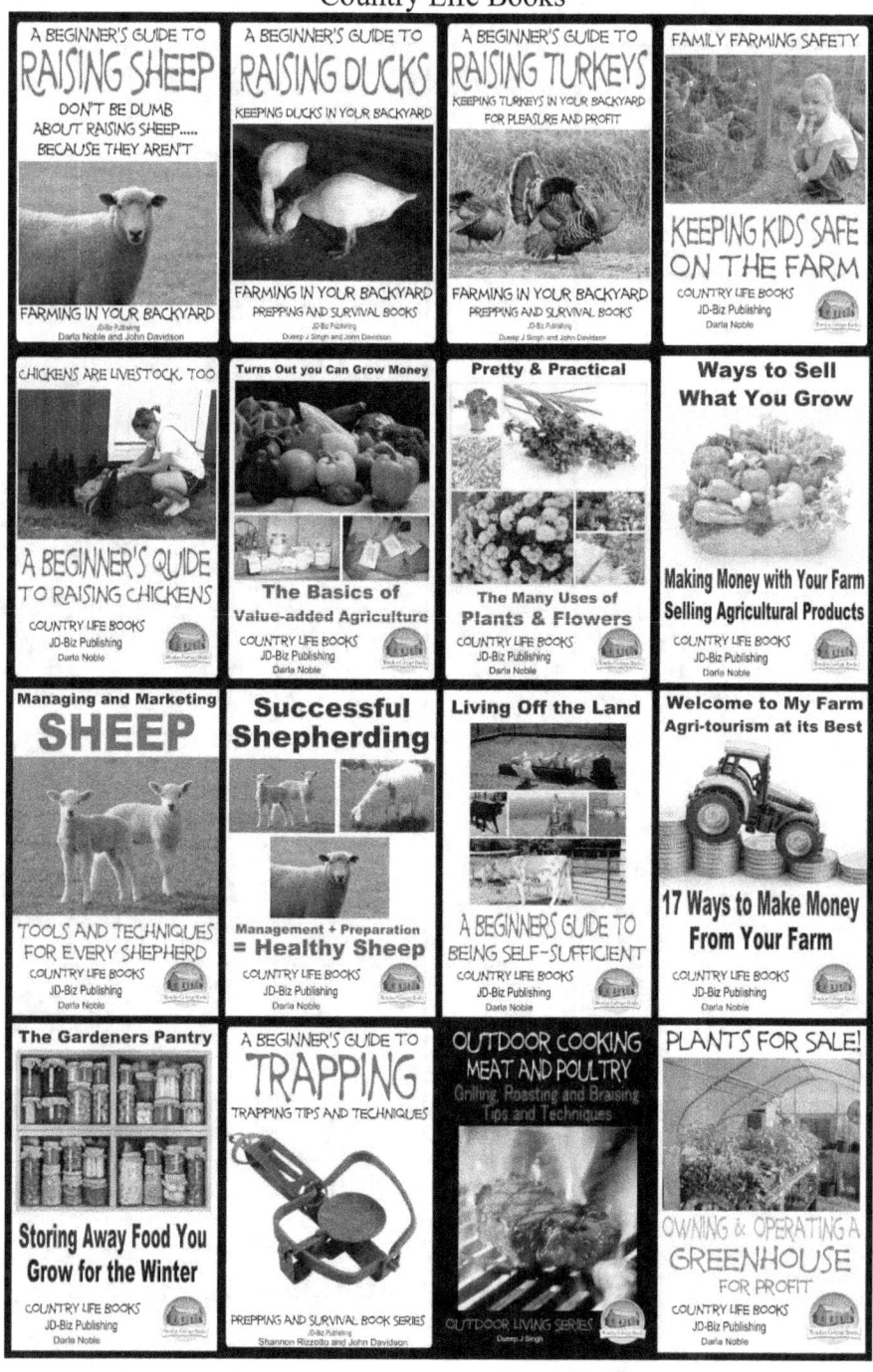

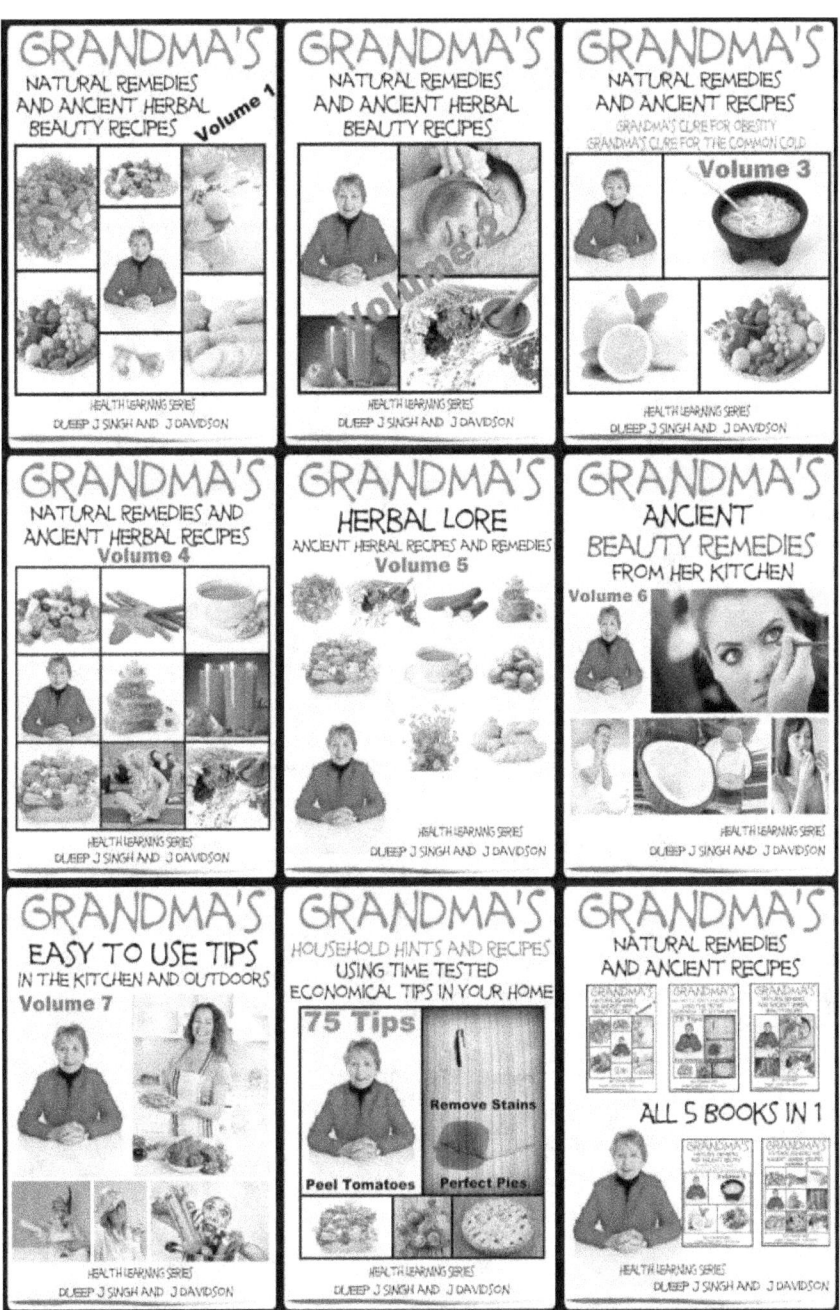

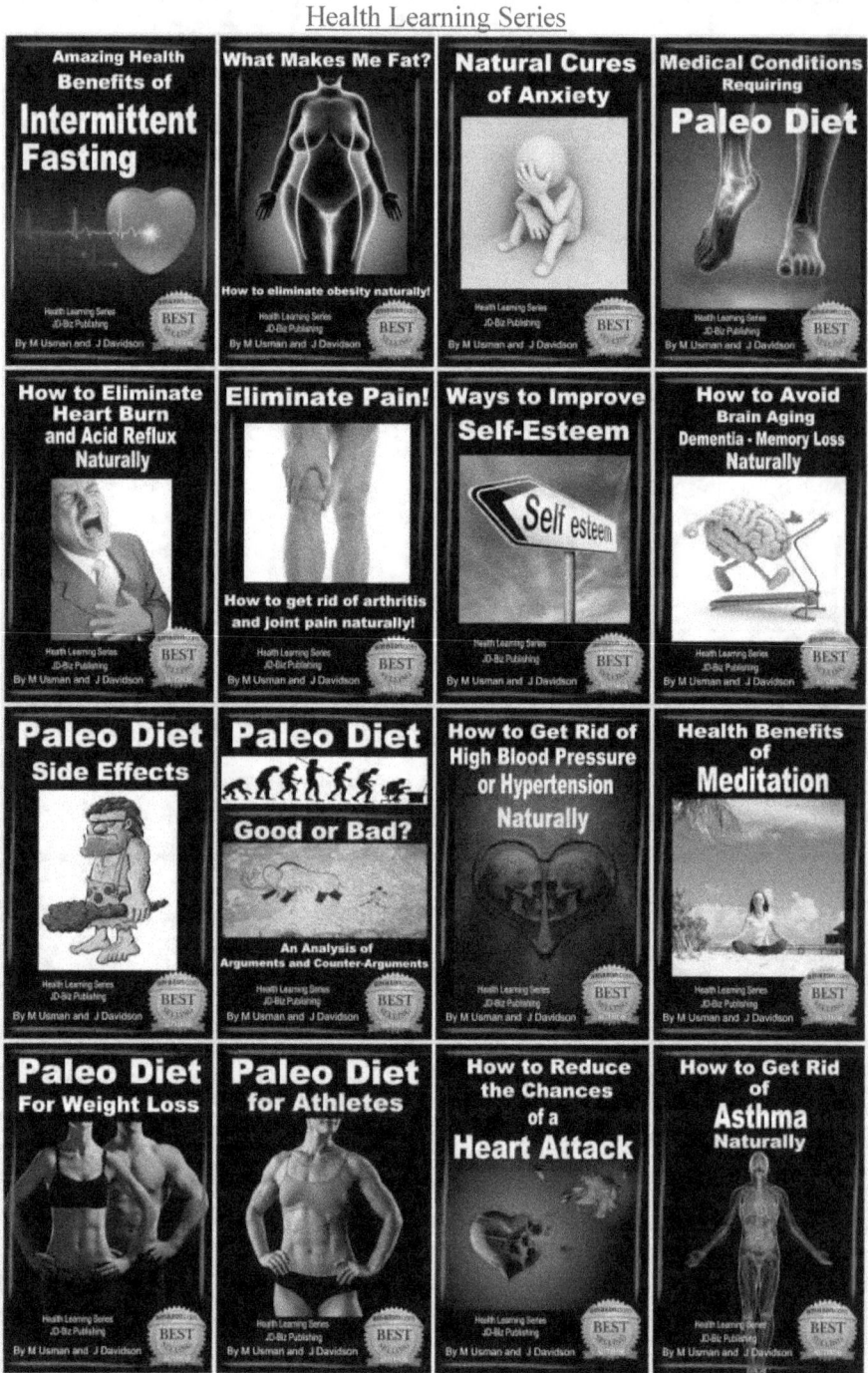

Amazing Animal Book Series

Learn To Draw Series

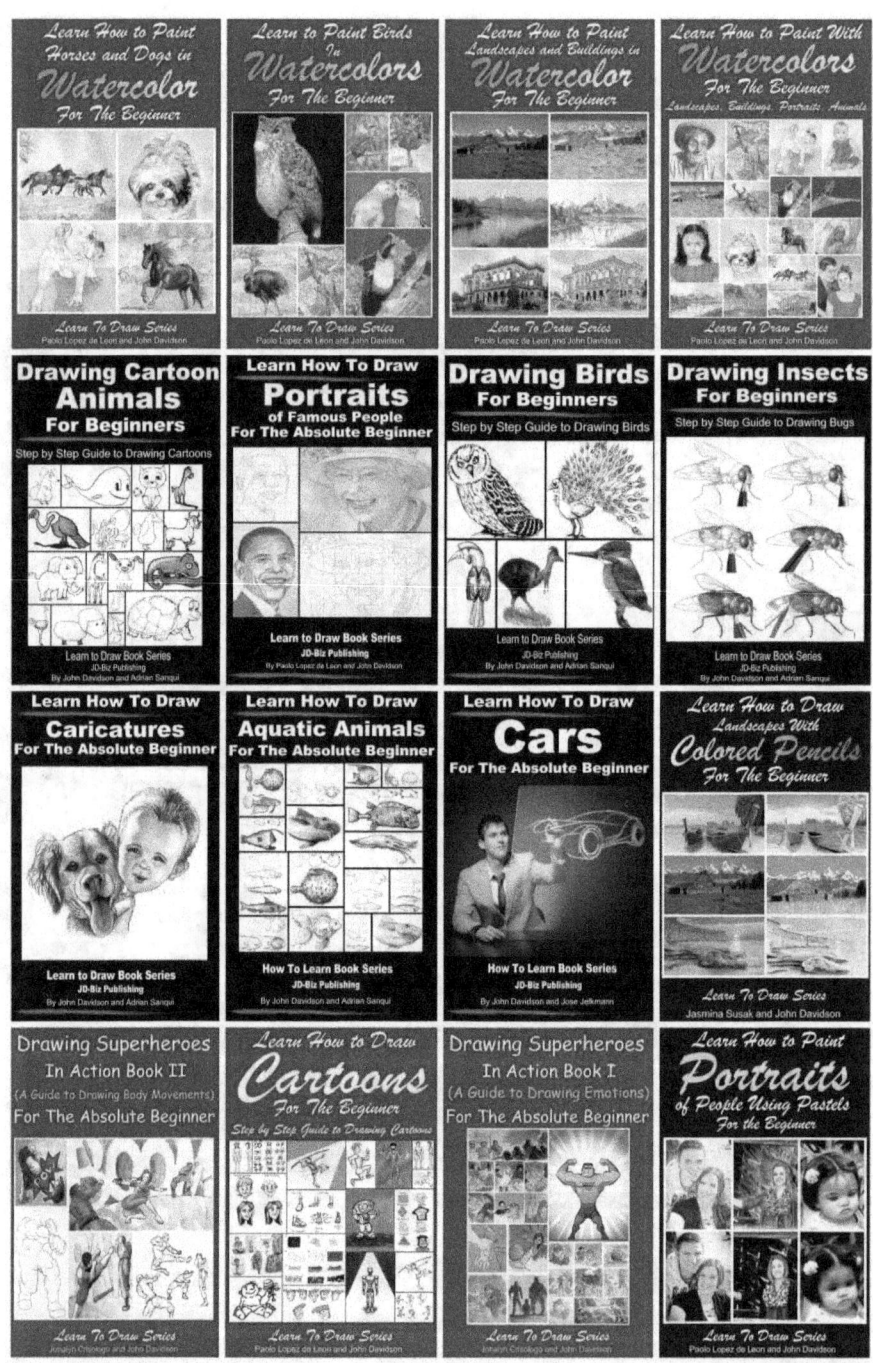

How to Build and Plan Books

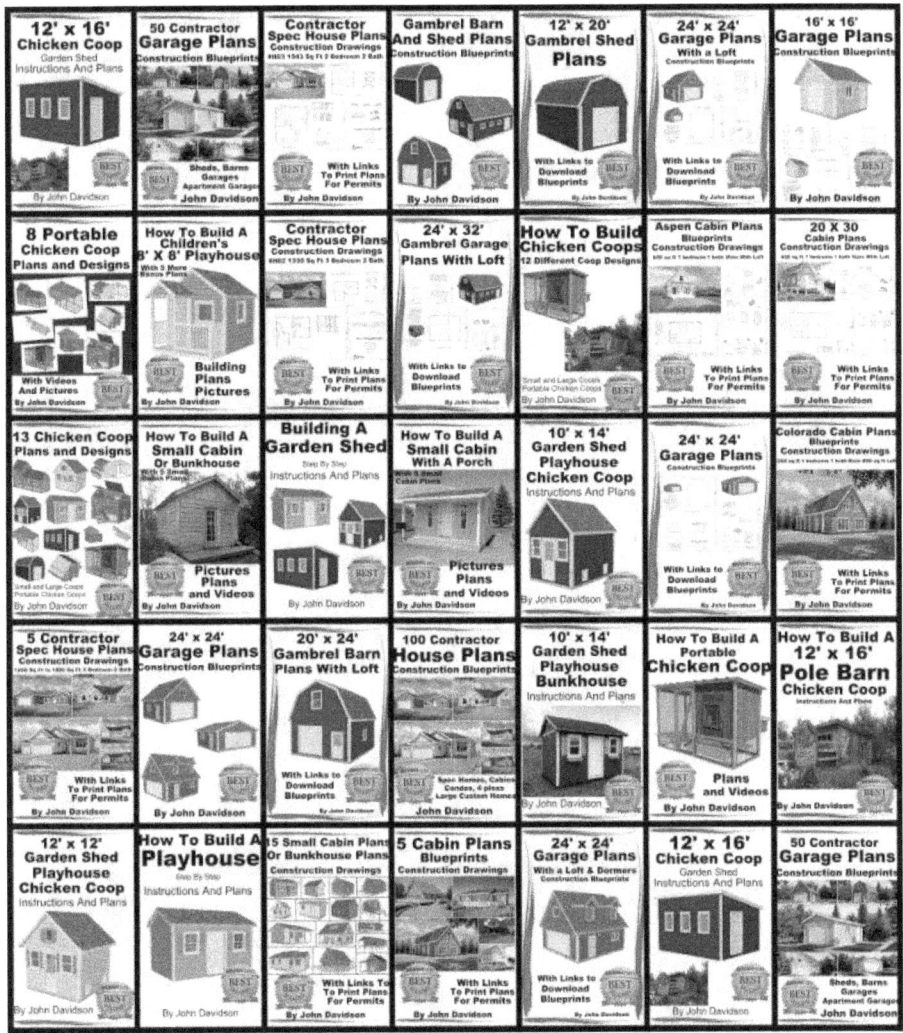

Entrepreneur Book Series

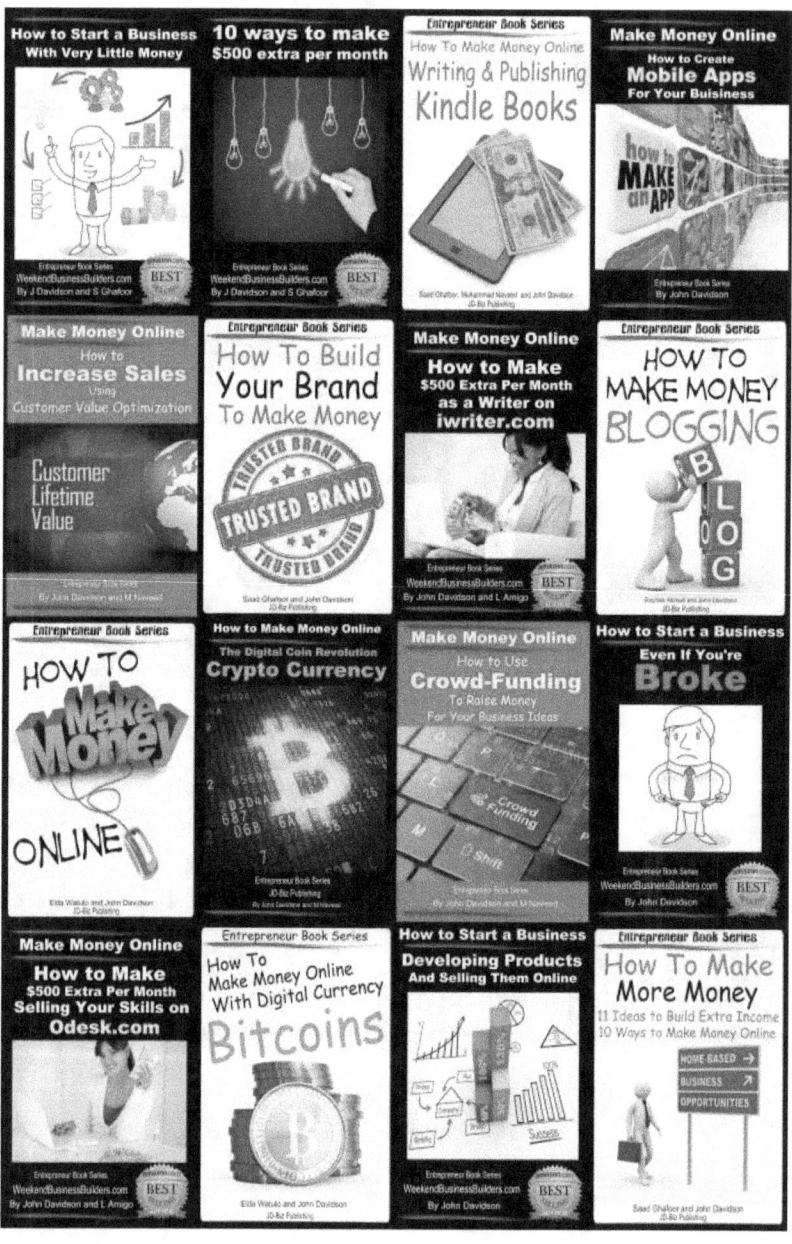

Our books are available at

1. Amazon.com

2. Barnes and Noble

3. Itunes

4. Kobo

5. Smashwords

6. Google Play Books

Publisher

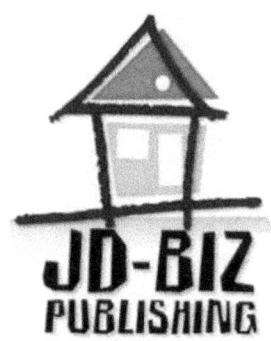

JD-Biz Corp

P O Box 374

Mendon, Utah 84325

http://www.jd-biz.com/

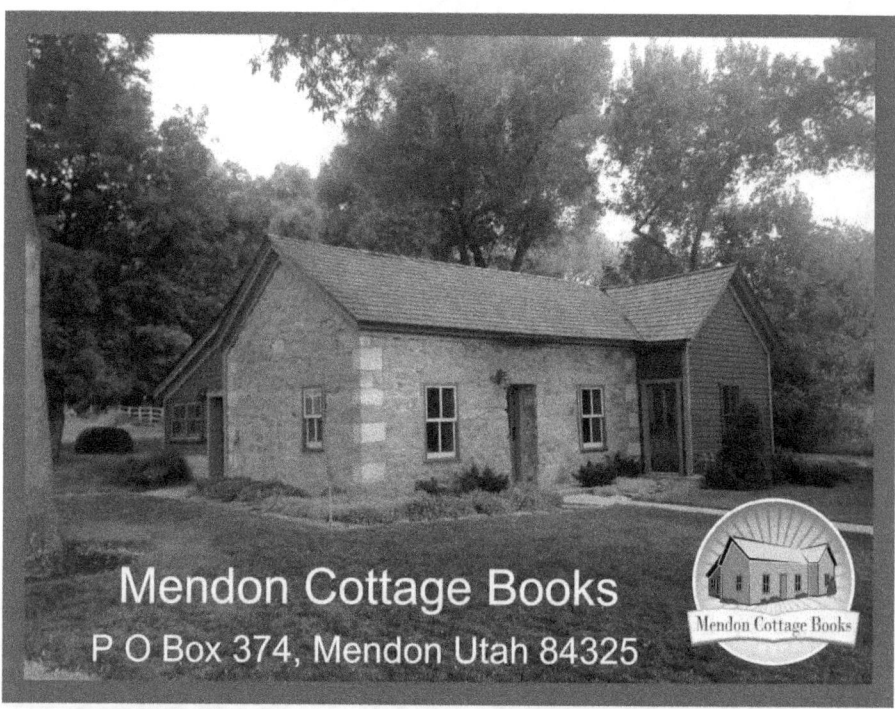